Communication and Swallowing Solutions for the ALS/MND Community

A CINI Manual

Communication and Swallowing Solutions for the ALS/MND Community

A CINI Manual

Edited by
Marta S. Kazandjian, M.A. CCC-SLP
Executive Director
Communication Independence
for the Neurologically
Impaired, Inc.

SINGULAR PUBLISHING GROUP, INC.
SAN DIEGO · LONDON

Singular Publishing Group, Inc.
401 West "A" Street, Suite 325
San Diego, California 92101-7904

19 Compton Terrace
London N1 2UN, U.K.

Typeset in 11/14 Bookman by So Cal Graphics
Printed in the United States of America by BookCrafters

Library of Congress Cataloging-in-Publication Data

Communication and swallowing solutions for the ALS/MND community : a CINI manual / ed., Marta S. Kazandjian
     p.   cm.
  ISBN 1-56593-808-9
  1. Speech disorders. 2. Deglutition disorders. 3. Amyotrophic lateral sclerosis—Complications   I. Kazandjian, Marta S.
II. Communication Independence for the Neurologically Impaired, Inc.
  [DNLM: 1. Amyotrophic Lateral Sclerosis—rehabilitation. 2. Motor Neuron Diseases—rehabilitation. 3. Speech Disorders—
rehabilitation. 4. Deglutition Disorders—rehabilitation. WE 550
C734 1996]
RC423.C627   1996
616.8'3—dc20
                                            96-32631
                                            CIP

Contents

This section is devoted to a general overview of
ALS/MND, defining pseudobulbar palsy, how
ALS/MND affects communication and swallowing, and
ALS/MND as a progressive neuromuscular disease.

This section reviews the role of the speech-language
pathologist and augmentative communication systems.
It provides information on working with your speech-
language pathologist and augmentative
communication team to select the most appropriate
communication system. Issues such as funding are
discussed. It also covers topics such as
communication by telephone, the use of switches, and
the use of electronic systems to communicate with
other patients with ALS/MND. This section also
discusses tracheostomy and ventilator dependence.

This section defines dysphagia (swallowing
impairment). It reviews the normal swallowing process,
how ALS/MND effects swallowing, and how swallowing
function is tested. It describes how the speech-

language pathologist helps the patient learn compensatory swallowing techniques to facilitate safe swallowing. Saliva control and dietary changes are reviewed as well as alternative feeding methods, if eating by mouth is no longer possible.

Preface

Amyotrophic lateral sclerosis (ALS), also known as *Lou Gehrig's disease* or *Motor neuron disease (MND)*, is a disease frightening to a patient, family, and friends. Although our prayers are for a cure, we must still deal with the ongoing deterioration to the muscles caused by the disease and the effect this has on the quality of a patient's life. For the first time there are new developments that offer a glimmer of hope to those afflicted by this dreadful disease.

The professionals of Communication Independence for the Neurologically Impaired (CINI) have come together with the intention of creating a resource manual. Our purpose is to lead patients, families, and medical professionals through the stages of managing communication and swallowing impairment created during various stages of ALS/ MND. Our desire is to provide ALS/MND patients and caregivers with the knowledge and experience of our professional staff and to help those afflicted to maintain the highest possible quality of life. This manual will provide some insight into the many options available to solve communication and swallowing problems as they arise and illustrate how these solutions can be used to support and resolve a patient's needs.

As professionals who have assisted patients and families for many years, we believe a written manual is the most effective means to alert everyone to both the problems and potential solutions that accompany a loss of communication and swallowing. This manual begins the educational process that will help patients, families, and medical professionals take an *active* role in managing the disease. We provide readers with a description of potential intervention techniques and the role that each medical professional takes in managing the disease.

For many, the solutions to the problems caused by the loss of the ability to speak and swallow will be almost as frightening as the disease, itself, because these solutions involve technology. We can only assure you that we have many patients who have used the solutions presented here with great success and effectiveness. Many of them lead active lives and continue to contribute to their family, friends, and community.

Losing the ability to communicate can be very disheartening. Without the ability to communicate, one loses his or her ability to direct their own care, make personal decisions, and function in today's environment. Learning new ways to express one's ideas and thoughts can be challenging and rewarding. CINI's greatest challenge is to assist patients in maintaining the highest level of communication possible. Maximizing communication function assists a person in preserving quality of life and independence and maintenance of dignity.

We hope that this resource manual provides persons with ALS/MND, caregivers and families with the necessary information to ask questions and make informed decisions to best manage communication and swallowing difficulties.

Acknowledgments

Communication Independence for the Neurologically Impaired's (CINI) inception resulted from a discussion of a dream. What could be done to assist patients who are diagnosed with neurological diseases to continue to communicate throughout the course of their disease? How can patients be better educated to inquire and seek the guidance of health care professionals who can facilitate this process? These questions began CINI's mission. Through the dedication and support of many people, CINI has begun to provide some answers for communicatively impaired patients.

The commitment to this mission is no better illustrated than by Peter Strugatz, CINI's Co-Founder and President, who turned the concept of CINI into a reality. Peter experienced the devastation of neurological disease as his mother lived through the stages of ALS. He came to understand how communication and true quality of life in the neurologically impaired patient are inseparable.

I would like to thank the many people who joined our team to develop CINI during its formative stages and who assisted in the completion of this resource manual. Thank you to Lisa Adams, M.A., CCC, who spent many painstaking hours researching and writing about the augmentative communication evaluation process; to Karen Dikeman, M.A., CCC for sharing her expertise in swallowing management; to Frima Christopher, Ph.D., for giving us insight into the emotional roller coaster that our patients and caregivers experience; to Joel Delfiner, M.D., for sharing his knowledge in managing the neurologically impaired patient; and to Mr. Walter Green for the hours he spent in assisting us, not only in CINI's growth, but for providing the patient perspective.

I would also like to thank Donna King, CINI's Administrative Manager, for her patience and commitment not only to CINI's patients but to making the resource manual manuscript user friendly; to Donna Strugatz, Esq., for her special projects work in legal and business affairs; to Seth Perlman, Esq., CINI's attorney, for his advice and time; and, many thanks to Gregory Butterick who fielded and continues to field our technology, computer-related questions.

This resource manual was accomplished with a team effort. I hope that this will be the first of CINI's commitment to making communication possible for the neurologically impaired.

Marta Kazandjian, M.A., CCC
Speech-Language Pathologist
Co-Founder, Executive Director, CINI

CINI

(Communication Independence for the Neurologically Impaired)

Communication of our feelings, needs, and intentions is the essence of being human. For many neurologically impaired individuals, however, the loss of the ability to communicate through the spoken or written word is a devastating and frustrating reality.

Some professionals who work with the ALS/MND population have come together to establish Communication Independence for the Neurologically Impaired (CINI). CINI's primary goal is to provide augmentative communication information and services to those patients who may be unable to obtain evaluation and treatment at established communication centers.

CINI's aim is to be a resource for patients, families, caregivers, and professionals by providing necessary information about communication and swallowing. This ensures that the patient with ALS/MND is fully aware of all the management options available. The patient will have the knowledge to participate more effectively in decision making and to obtain services to facilitate communication and swallowing through the course of the disease. This manual is the work of the professionals of CINI.

For more information about Communication Independence for the Neurologically Impaired, Inc., contact us at:

CINI
250 Mercer Street, Suite B1608
New York, NY 10012

Telephone: (516) 874-8354
Fax: (516) 878-8412
Internet Address: 73523.151@CompuServe.com
CompuServe Address: 73523,151
Prodigy Address: UYLR96A

Additional information about CINI can be found on our Web Site. The address of our Web Site is:
http://www.cini.org

CINI is a 501c (3) nonprofit corporation.

What Is Amyotrophic Lateral Sclerosis/Motor Neuron Disease?

This section is divided into a series of questions to assist you with ALS/MND in understanding the nature and effect ALS/MND has on patients.

What is ALS/MND: Lou Gehrig's Disease?

Amyotrophic lateral sclerosis (ALS), used synonomously with *Motor neuron disease* or *Lou Gehrig's disease* (MND), is a neuromuscular disease that results in the deterioration of muscles throughout the body. This muscle deterioration occurs because the nerves stemming from the brain and spinal cord are damaged from the disease process. The disease affects 30,000 people per year just in the United States, with approximately 5,000 new cases diagnosed annually. Although progressive deterioration is characteristic of the disease, mental capacity or cognition is rarely affected. The cause of ALS/MND is still unknown. Although important new information has been recently obtained from drug trials and research studies, a cure has not yet been found.

ALS/MND can present and progress in a variety of ways. Specialists in this area have classified the disorders by several different methods. One traditional classification scheme uses the observable physical signs of the illness to describe the conditions.

Classical ALS/MND produces weakness, loss of muscle bulk, abnormal muscle twitches (fasciculations), abnormal muscle stiffness (spasticity), and overactive muscle tendon reflexes. Any muscle under voluntary control can be affected, including the arm muscles, leg muscles, muscles of speaking, muscles of swallowing, and muscles of breathing. The illness usually begins in one region of the body (e.g., one arm or the mouth and throat), but eventually can spread to other regions.

Progressive bulbar palsy (*PBP*) results in progressive weakness and atrophy of the muscles of swallowing, speaking, and, eventually, breathing. The tongue muscle wastes away and may appear to continually twitch. There is no true weakness in the arms or legs, but the muscle tendon reflexes may be overactive.

Progressive muscular atrophy (*PMA*) is similar to classic ALS/MND, except that there is no muscle stiffness and the muscle tendon reflexes are reduced or absent.

Primary lateral sclerosis (*PLS*) produces progressive stiffness and weakness of the muscles without loss of muscle bulk and without fasciculations. The muscle tendon reflexes are extremely overactive. Speech and swallowing can be affected.

My doctor used the term "pseudobulbar palsy." What does that mean? Is it part of ALS/MND?

The term "pseudobulbar palsy" describes a condition in which there is impaired speaking and swallowing due to stiffness and spasticity of the relevant muscles, but no loss of muscle bulk. This can be seen in classic ALS/MND, PBP, and PLS. One unusual feature of this condition is inappropriate laughter and crying. An individual with this condition will laugh at minimally amusing situations or cry when not really sad. People afflicted with this are not psychiatrically impaired and are not senile. They are aware of the inappropriateness of this response, but cannot control it because of damage to specific brain structures and pathways.

How can ALS/MND affect communication and swallowing?

Not all individuals affected with ALS/MND have speech and swallowing problems; however, in some cases, the impact of the disease on communication and swallowing can be devastating. For those who do have speech and swallowing problems, there are professionals who are skilled in working with these patients and are able to provide access to a communication method, even when spoken output is no longer possible. These professionals can also assist in facilitating safe swallowing for longer periods of time. With the assistance of these professionals, those afflicted with ALS/MND can maintain independence, decision making ability, and control over their lives.

Sometimes, slurred speech or difficulty swallowing is the first sign of ALS/MND. The slurred articulation may worsen until the patient is poorly understood even by listeners they know well. Eventually, the ability to move the speech muscles, especially the tongue, may become severely reduced, and the patient is no longer able to use speech as a functional method for message transfer or communication. At some time during this deterioration, a special method of communication known as augmentative or alternative communication may be prescribed. For some individuals, the muscles of breathing may also become impaired. If a patient becomes weak and cannot breathe adequately on his or her own, some type of assisted ventilation may be prescribed by the doctor. Mechanical ventilation may interfere with speech and swallowing. The speech-language pathologist (SLP) can assist an individual in maximizing communication and swallowing in this situation.

A patient's swallowing function may deteriorate in a similar progression. Various consistencies of food may slowly become more difficult to manage. As swallowing status decreases, eating safely by mouth becomes a problem. At this time the physician may recommend an alternative method of feeding.

If ALS/MND is a progressive disease and there is no cure, what can we do?

At the time of the diagnosis, the individual is often told that ALS/MND is a progressive neuromuscular disease for which there is no cure. However, that there is no cure for ALS/MND does *not* mean that a patient cannot be helped.

As stated previously, the progression of ALS/MND is not the same for one individual as for another. Despite the unpredictability of the disease, patients can educate themselves about the many ways their bodies may be affected. The earlier a patient learns about the process of the disease, the more effective he or she can be in preempting potential problems. The concept of preempting problems means that he or she has ways to manage difficult problems before they become a major source of concern. One example of this can be in swallowing. The patient should know in advance that swallowing function may deteriorate. When the initial muscle weakness is noted, the patient should consult with a speech-language pathologist (SLP) and dietician. These professionals will assist the individual in modifying his or her diet by selecting and preparing foods that will be easier to swallow. Another example of preempting a problem may include the purchase of a computer for eventual communication use. The patient should be helped by the speech-language pathologist in developing a system that will be useful through all stages of the disease—even late stages.

It is essential that both patients and caregivers seek the help of trained health care professionals early in the disease process. This will enable them to preempt problems before they become critical. The health care professionals may call on each other to assist in maximizing various body functions to maintain the highest possible quality of life.

Maintenance is a key concept in managing a disease like ALS/MND. Patients can help maintain function by exercising and continuing to use their muscles. For example, many individuals follow a program of occupational and physical therapy that includes exercises for the arms, legs, hands, and chest. The speech-language pathologist will suggest exercise for the muscles of the face and mouth. Compensatory strategies may be suggested by health care professionals to support the decreased function that occurs as the disease progresses.

When the muscle weakness increases, therapists may suggest alternative methods of communicating, moving, or eating. These methods often involve the use of electronic equipment. For example, a patient whose speech has become very difficult to understand may choose to communicate chiefly via a computer with voice output capacity.

Patients and caregivers must educate themselves about the many services offered by health care professionals. Education allows intelligent choices to be made in the selection of the appropriate health care services. Additionally, the patient will be able to self-direct care more effectively and get what is needed when equipped with knowledge. This, in turn, allows the health care team to better meet the patient's needs.

When a patient has an understanding of the disease process, plans can be made to address each need. The team of patient and health care professionals can then be proactive in the management of the disease. Problems can be anticipated and solutions can be waiting to fill these needs as they happen. The greater the degree of readiness a patient and his or her caregiver has, the less they will be overwhelmed by the various stages of the disease.

Communication Intervention

This section is divided into a series of questions to help patients with ALS/MND in understanding how to address communication problems in ALS/MND.

(continued)

What is the role of the speech-language pathologist (SLP) in managing communication impairments of patients with ALS/MND?

The muscles for speech and swallowing may possibly be affected by ALS/MND. The speech-language pathologist (SLP) can help by providing strategies to maintain spoken speech for as long as possible. Initial intervention strategies may include oral exercises to maintain the range of motion and strength of the mouth including the tongue, lips, and jaw. Techniques to maximize the way that speech sounds are understood are also introduced. The patient is taught to slow speech and exaggerate each word to compensate for slurred speech. If the ability to speak loudly decreases, an amplifier can be used to increase loudness for better listener comprehension.

What is an augmentative communication system?

An augmentative/alternative communication system (ACS) allows for communication, even when an individual's speech is not well understood. An augmentative communication system (ACS) does not have to be a computer, although some augmentative communication systems are designed with computerized elements. The decision to use an ACS is very individual. Although an ACS is generally used by patients who cannot speak, it may also be used by patients who are beginning to have trouble speaking or writing. For example, the individual who is understood by family members but not by strangers may consider an augmentative communication system to "augment" message transfer and exchange. This may include spelling the beginning of a word or providing the first few letters as a cue to a word that is being spoken.

Ideally, an augmentative communication system should provide a reliable, consistent, and easy-to-use method of communication. The patient can expect the SLP to determine what is needed during an evaluation and to assist in selecting and developing an optimal ACS.

What is the role of the speech-language pathologist in acquiring an augmentative communication system?

The SLP is responsible for evaluating the patient for an augmentative communication system and for teaching the patient with ALS/MND to use the system for communication.

How do I find a qualified speech-language pathologist?

The American Speech Language and Hearing Association (ASHA) is the national association of speech-language pathologists in the United States. It provides information about practicing clinicians in each state. Within this association is a special interest division for augmentative communication. This division is a smaller number of speech pathologists with a special interest in augmentative communication. ASHA can provide you with names of speech-language pathologists who are part of this special interest division in your state (see Appendix B).

The United States Society of Alternative and Augmentative Communication (USSAAC) is another national association that represents speech-language pathologists who have a special interest in augmentative communication. This national and the international organization International Society of Alternative and Augmentative Communication (ISAAC) can be contacted for a referral (see Appendix B).

When contacting a speech-language pathologist, you should ask the clinician if she or he has experience in working with assistive devices and augmentative communication systems. This is considered a specialty area for clinicians and, therefore, may not be the expertise of all speech-language pathologists.

What takes place during the communication evaluation process?

An augmentative communication evaluation can be performed in a hospital, a clinic, an office, or the home. It must be performed by a licensed speech-language pathologist. The SLP experienced in working with ALS/MND understands that the patient has a disease that progressively deteriorates and weakens the body. An awareness of this is essential when choosing an ACS, because communication skills demonstrated during evaluation, such as writing or typing, may become weaker or nonfunctional in the future. The individual must always be able to operate the ACS despite possible future deterioration of the body.

During or after an evaluation, the SLP may request advice from other rehabilitation professionals, including the occupational therapist or physical therapist, working with an individual. These professionals assist the SLP in specialized ways, such as improving the patient's seating and positioning in a chair, bed, or wheelchair. They may also fit a person with splints or other adaptive devices. A splint is a support device used by occupational and physical therapists to help maintain a hand, arm, or leg in a given position. When limb muscles are weak, they often contract, which can lead to contractures, or muscle shortening. A splint can help to avoid contractures of weak extremities. Such participation of more than one professional is an aspect of what is called a *team approach* and is highly recommended for a thorough evaluation.

The SLP will evaluate each of the following areas during the augmentative communication evaluation.

The Case History

The SLP first takes a case history from the patient. This case history includes the approximate date of onset of the disease, the name of the primary care physician (usually a neurologist or internist), and the name of the hospital where the individual receives treatment. The SLP will ask about services received from other health care professionals, including home health aid, occupational therapist, physical therapist, and respiratory therapist. The SLP will also take a medical case history that includes questions about previous neurological problems (i.e., stroke), episodes of pneumonia, and so on. Finally, the SLP will take information about the patient's family, as well as social and professional life to help understand all the communication needs of the individual.

Speech

The SLP will assess the degree to which speech has been affected by the disease. The loss of speech due to weakening of the musculature is known as dysarthria. In some cases, the muscle deterioration can ultimately progress until the patient has no speech left. This condition is called anarthria. The SLP will observe the patient communicating with significant others to determine how successful speech is as a method of communication. Often, the husband, wife, or child of the individual will continue to understand the patient's speech long after persons less familiar with the individual have ceased to understand. An ACS may be necessary in special situations to supplement or "augment" speech (e.g., interacting with a server at a restaurant) and unaided speech may continue to be useful in other situations (e.g., at home with family).

Language

Language is a person's ability to combine words into sentences to communicate ideas. A person who cannot speak may do this through writing. The SLP assesses the language ability of the patient to determine its status. ALS/MND does not usually alter a person's ability to use language, and this section of the evaluation is usually brief. However, there are certain neurological injuries that can affect a person's ability to use language normally. The language assessment will be conducted in the patient's native language. Language assessment includes literacy. If an individual is not literate (never learned to read or write), the SLP can design an ACS that does not involve letters and words, but may utilize pictures or symbols to represent things, ideas, and meaning.

Vision

As most ACS rely on a person's ability to see a chart, notebook, or screen, the SLP will ask the patient questions about vision during the evaluation. The patient should have his or her glasses available during the evaluation. If vision is seriously impaired (i.e., from low vision or cataracts) or if the individual is blind, the SLP should be informed of this prior to the evaluation so the necessary provisions can be made to adapt the evaluation procedures.

Physical Motor

One of the most important areas of assessment is physical motor capability. Physical motor capability means the motor movements that are available to the patient. These will change during various stages of the disease process. Physical motor deterioration is highly variable from individual to individual. One patient may lose speech but continue to be able to move his or her hands; another patient may be able to talk but have little movement in the arms and legs.

The SLP evaluates all parts of the body to determine which movements are available. This includes large muscle movements such as head turning as well as small muscle movements such as lifting the eyebrow or twitching a finger or cheek. It is important to remember that, as ALS/MND is a progressive disease, the movements that the SLP identifies may not be available to the patient in the near or distant future. For this reason, physical motor capability needs to be constantly reevaluated.

Even though I can't move my hands to write or type, will I still be able to operate a communication system?

Patients often operate even sophisticated computers without using their hands. Once the evaluation process is complete, the SLP will consider the findings and present options for various communication systems for each patient. The options that will be presented by the SLP will result from all parts of the evaluation; however, decisions are most heavily influenced by the physical motor capabilities of an individual. If muscles for speech are no longer functional, the patients will need to use another part of the body for communication. The SLP identifies the part of the body that the individual can best control. For one patient, movement of the hands may be easiest, although for another it may be movement of a finger, and for another it may be movement of the eyes. The most important factor in identifying this motor movement is that the movement pattern be easy, reliable, and consistently available to the individual. If the movement pattern is tiring or unreliable, the individual will not be able to use it consistently for communication throughout the day. Often, an occupational therapist or physical therapist assists the SLP in identifying this movement pattern. This is part of the team approach to treatment.

During the evaluation I heard the term "access method." What does this mean?

Based on the information about physical motor capability, a method for *access* can be identified. The term access refers to the way the individual will operate the communication system. For example, one individual may use fingers for typing, with another moving the eyes to point at letters, thereby spelling words. An access method for an individual will often change as the disease progressively leads to weakening of different areas of the body. This means that a patient who at one point uses hands for communication may lose this ability and eventually have to use another access method. It is important for each individual to know that communication does not have to stop simply because hands become weak and typing is no longer possible. A variety of access methods are available to extend communication.

What are examples of access methods that I can use?

Access methods can range from a simple, nonelectronic communication system to an electronic, computer-based communication system. Maintaining communication allows the patient to continue to manage his or her life. Each method of access allows the patient to communicate despite physical motor weakness. The following are possible access methods:

Pencil and Paper Writing

Because ALS/MND affects people in different ways, the loss of speech may occur before other parts of the body weaken. These patients often use writing as a form of communication. If the clarity of speech is mildly to moderately impaired, the individual may use writing on occasions when talking to someone unfamiliar with him or her (e.g., a clerk in the grocery store). If speech is severely impaired, he or she may need to use writing all the time.

Over time, ALS/MND may weaken the hands of a patient who has used writing as a form of communication. The SLP, in combination with an occupational therapist (OT), may then explore ways to prolong the ability to write, despite the weakness. Sometimes, if the individual's grip on a pen is loose, a "built-up" pen (a pen wrapped in foam or cloth to thicken the width) can be used. Additionally, the OT may develop a splint or a device for anchoring the pen to the hand, which alleviates the need to grasp the pen. It is important to explore all options for maintaining the capacity to write with the assistance of augmentative communication specialists before moving to another access method.

Direct Selection

Direct selection is best described as pointing directly at words, letters, or symbols. Although one automatically thinks of pointing with a finger, there are other methods for pointing.

An individual who can use a finger, but who can no longer hold a pen for writing, may elect to spell messages by pointing to letters on an alphabet board. The SLP in combination with an OT may assist the patient with pointing by using splints to keep the finger extended outward, or by using adaptive devices to make it easier for the patient to move the hand around an alphabet board.

Scanning

Scanning is an access method that is appropriate for individuals who have small motor movements remaining. If the ability to point using the hands is lost, a patient can use a part of the body to "signal" the communication partner. The signal may be raising the finger, the eyebrows, or the eyes or twitching a certain muscle in the body, for example on the arm or face. This signal allows the individual to control the communication system. This is done by presenting items one at a time to the individual. For the patient with ALS/MND, these items are usually letters of the alphabet. The patient signals when the desired letter is presented. The communication partner writes down each letter until the message is complete. One example of scanning is illustrated in Figure 1. Because only small motor movements are required, the patient can continue to use scanning systems even as the disease progresses. There are many patients who use eye blinks as a scanning signal with great success.

Eyegaze

Eyegaze is actually a form of direct selection, because the eyes are responsible for "pointing" at words, letters, or symbols, as illustrated in Figure 2. Eyegaze systems are an

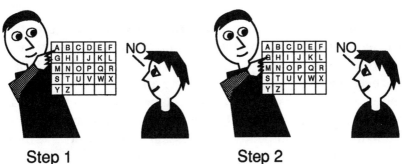

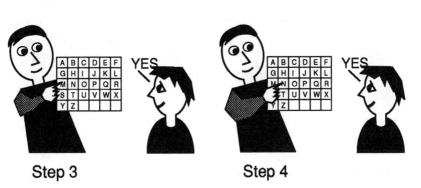

Figure 1. An example of row-column scanning (Adapted from *Electronic Communication Aids, Selection and Use* by I. Fishman, 1987, p. 71. San Diego: College-Hill Press. Copyright by I. Fishman)

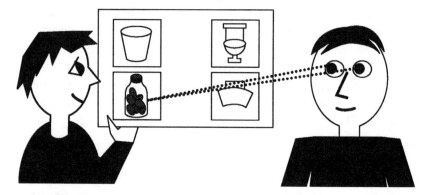

Figure 2. Direct selection through eyegaze. (From *Communication and Swallowing Management of Tracheostomized and Ventilator Dependent Adults* by K. Dikeman and M. Kazandjian, 1995, p. 211. San Diego: Singular Publishing Group.)

excellent choice for many patients, because movement of the eyes and eyelids usually remain relatively strong, even as the disease weakens other parts of the body. Additionally, because the patient is pointing directly at the desired letter, communication is accomplished more rapidly than with a scanning system. However, eyegaze systems are more difficult to learn for both the message sender and the message receiver. A commonly used eyegaze system is called an Eye-Link. Letters of the alphabet are organized on a piece of clear plastic. The listener holds this clear alphabet board toward the individual. The individual looks at each letter of the message. The listener watches the individual's eyes and deciphers the letter. Each letter is selected until the message is complete. Figure 3 illustrates instructions for use of an Eye-Link.

Coded Systems

With a coded system, the patient learns a "code," which is then deciphered by the listener. This code is usually a combination of some sort, which stands for message

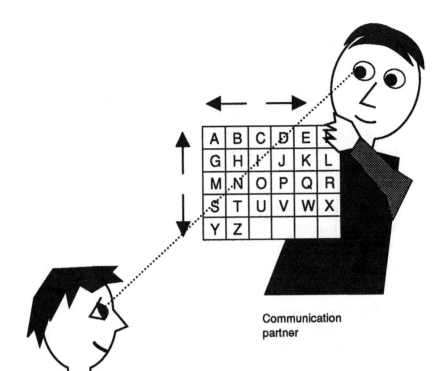

Communication partner

Patient

1. Hold sheet in front of the patient
2. Have patient focus on the first letter of the word desired
3. Move sheet until your eyes "link" with the patient's through the desired letter
4. Check with the patient to see if you are correct
5. Continue the process until you get the message

Figure 3. Instructions for use of an Eye-link. (Reprinted from *Communication and Swallowing Management of Tracheostomized and Ventilator Dependent Adults* by K. Dikeman and M. Kazandjian, 1995, p. 211. San Diego: Singular Publishing Group, with permission.)

units, such as letters of the alphabet or words and phrases. An E-Tran can be used to communicate messages via a coded system. For example, "C-1" can be used to stand for "please reposition me" as is illustrated in Figure 4. Time is saved by using the brief code to represent a longer message. A coded system is selected when the individual wants access to a large amount of language, but does not have the motor control to point to all the items. The most commonly used coded system for patients is Morse code. The individual using Morse code may be able to use small motor movements to activate a buzzer system. The combination of buzzes is then converted to letters of the alphabet. Morse code is especially effective when using a computer.

What is a nonelectronic communication system and how does it differ from an electronic communication system?

Nonelectronic communication systems are tailor-made for each individual user and are not electronically operated. An example is a written letterboard containing letters, words, and phrases. Nonelectronic communication systems have the advantage of being inexpensive, readily available, highly portable, and resistant to breakage. They are excellent backup systems for those when an electronic system is not functioning. However, many communication needs cannot be met with these nonelectronic communication systems.

A nonelectronic communication system requires that the listener be close to the patient to receive the message. Sometimes, as with a scanning system, the listener must assist the individual in sending the message by presenting letters of the alphabet. If no trained assistant is available to help, the message cannot be transmitted. This limits the individual's important communication independence. Additionally,

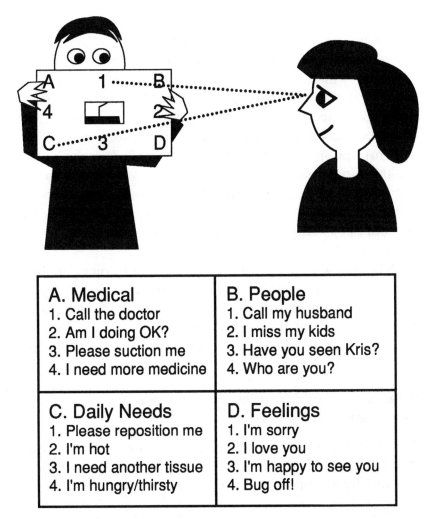

Figure 4. A coded system through the use of an E-Tran. (From *Communication and Swallowing Management of Tracheostomized and Ventilator Dependent Adults* by K. Dikeman and M. Kazandjian, 1995, p. 215. San Diego: Singular Publishing Group, with permission.)

a nonelectronic system cannot produce written output, which is also called hard copy. This means that a listener must always be present and that messages cannot be prepared in advance for later use.

Electronic communication devices can offer the patient increased independence in a variety of ways. Some electronic communication devices come with synthetic voice capacity, which allows the individual to "speak" a message. This eliminates the need for the listener to be physically close to the individual during communicative exchanges. Electronic communication devices may come with an option to produce written output, thereby allowing the individual to prepare messages in advance with a high degree of independence. Sending messages through electronic mail, faxes, and voice output (i.e., synthesized speech) are examples of other electronic solutions.

Individuals who use augmentative communication systems ideally have both a nonelectronic and an electronic communication system. The patient should discuss combining the use of the nonelectronic and electronic communication systems with the SLP during the evaluation.

What are some examples of nonelectronic communication systems?

The following are some frequently used nonelectronic communication systems. The choice of one of these systems is dictated by an individual's physical motor capabilities.

Writing

Writing in any form is the most readily available and portable method of communication. Writing does not have to involve pen and paper. It can be done on a chalkboard or a child's "Magic Slate" that permits the individual to write and then pull up the sheet to make the words disappear.

Alphabet Board

An alphabet board is simply a card that has the alphabet written on it from A to Z. The patient with ALS/MND points to the letters on this board and spells words for a listener. These boards can be made in a wide variety of sizes and may be designed to fit in a shirt pocket or purse. Words such as "thank-you" or phrases such as "I cannot speak, but I can spell" can be on the front or back of the board. Alphabet boards are often used by individuals who have speech that is difficult to understand. If the patient points to the first letter of a word while saying it, it helps the listener to understand that word more quickly and effectively. Figure 5 provides examples of alphabet and picture communication boards.

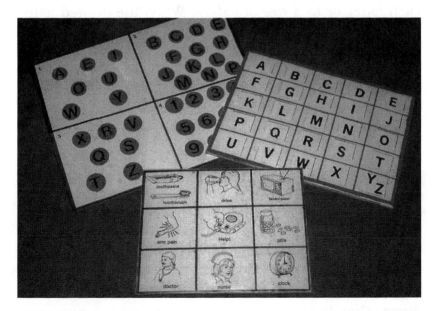

Figure 5. Examples of word, phrase, and picture communication boards. (From *Communication and Swallowing Management of Tracheostomized and Ventilator Dependent Adults* by K. Dikeman and M. Kazandjian, 1995, p. 210. San Diego: Singular Publishing Group, with permission.)

Communication Books

If the individual wants access to words he or she uses all the time (such as names), a combination word/phrase/alphabet book can be developed. For example, phrases such as "please reposition me" or "I'm thirsty" can be included. By making frequently used words available in such a book, the need to spell the same words over and over throughout the day can be alleviated.

Scanning Alphabet Board

A scanning alphabet board can be developed for individuals who cannot point to letters. The letters on an alphabet board are presented to the patient by the conversational partner. Usually the conversational partner will point to each letter or to a row of letters. When the desired letter is reached, the individual will raise his or her finger or eyes to signal "yes." Each letter is chosen until a word is spelled. As the patient becomes more experienced with this technique, a row of letters can be presented at a time so that the individual can spell more quickly.

Eye-Link

A clear plexiglass or plastic alphabet board can be developed for the patient to "look at" desired letters. The listener can stand across from the patient and identify the letters he or she looks at. This system is called an "Eye-Link." Eye-Links are commonly used by those who have severe physical motor impairments.

Phrase Boards

Some individuals find it helpful to make lists of frequently used phrases for communicating with a spouse, child, or nurse. These phrases are numbered for easy reference. The boards are then hung on the wall or in an easily accessible place. The patient need only say the number of the desired phrase, or the spouse or nurse can "scan" through the board until the desired phrase is reached.

The SLP should provide the patient with one or more of the above-mentioned communication systems. Despite the lure of a computerized communication device, non-electronic communication systems serve as readily available, inexpensive, reliable methods of communication.

What are some examples of electronic communication systems?

Many different electronic communication systems are available. The speech-language pathologist may help the patient try out several communication systems at the nearest evaluation center or in the patient's home. Some communication systems are custom designed for a specific user. Some communication systems offer symbols for users who are unable to spell. Communication systems can be designed to be used in specific situations, but are not efficient in providing communication throughout a day. For example, a communication system that works through a desktop computer cannot travel with the patient to doctor visits, but a laptop or notebook computer is more portable and will allow the patient to travel with the system. In selecting an electronic communication system, the individual must understand the features offered by the system and determine if those features best meet his or her needs. For example, individuals who have trouble seeing must select a system with a clear visual display. Most patients select a system that allows for spelling as opposed to symbols or pictures to represent a message.

A range of options are offered within various electronic communication devices. Some communication devices allow only one type of access (such as finger pointing or typing); other communication devices are designed to handle almost any type of access method, including direct selection, scanning, and coding. There are very few commercially available communication devices that will accept eyegaze as an input method. These systems are usually expensive. Research on eyegaze-operated communication devices is ongoing and may be a more affordable option in the future. It is best to select an electronic communication device that accepts a variety of access methods. As the disease progresses it may become necessary to move from one access method to another as a patient's physical motor function changes.

What are specific features that electronic communication systems may offer?

Electronic communication aids may be broken down into two broad groups: *Dedicated* electronic communication devices and *nondedicated* electronic communication devices. A dedicated device is built specifically for communication. A nondedicated device is built to perform other functions, but has been adapted to allow it to function for communication purposes. Personal and laptop computers fall into the category of nondedicated communication devices. Personal and laptop computers are designed to run all types of software. With the addition of certain accessories, they can run specialized software designed for individuals who are disabled.

In addition to these two broad distinctions, electronic communication systems can offer features that depend on patient needs and abilities. These features should be carefully considered according to individual needs. For example, for those who have problems with vision, the type of screen becomes a very important consideration. For some, it is essential to have a device that "speaks" and can be intelligible over the phone. For other patients, a speaking device is not essential, but a writing device is a requirement. These are choices that must be made by the individual afflicted with ALS/MND. They should not be made by anyone other than the patient who plans to use the device. Below are the most widely offered options:

Visual Display

The visual display is the screen or monitor on which the message appears. The size and clarity of the visual display can vary considerably from one device to the next. It is essential that the display meet the needs of a patient. It may be a small box or a full screen. Some communication devices have no visual display. Some displays have black writing on a gray background and may be difficult to see in direct sunlight because of glare. Communication devices can have a fluorescent display, usually green lettering on a black background which is easier to see. Most laptop personal computers contain liquid crystal displays (LCDs). These displays come in two styles: dual scan (often called DSTN) and active matrix (TFT) displays. Active matrix displays are sharper and clearer than the less expensive dual scan displays.

Voice Output

Many communication devices have voice output. Voice output may be in the form of synthesized speech or digitized speech. Synthesized speech is the most frequently used form of voice output. The sounds of the English language have been electronically synthesized so that any messages that the individual spells can be spoken by the communication device. The quality of synthesized speech varies widely. Poorly synthesized speech will sound robotic. Recent improvements in synthesized speech have a much more "human" tone. The quality of the synthesized speech affects the cost of the device. Synthesized speech is available in male or female voice. The patient controls the speed, pitch, and quality of the selected voice.

Digitized speech is a more sophisticated method of producing voice output that permits a much more "human" sounding speech. There are some electronic communication systems that combine a few minutes of digitized speech with synthesized speech. Most systems offering digitized speech limit the number of minutes that this speech is available for playback. A system may only offer 20 minutes of total recording time. Digitized speech is most often available in devices in which whole messages are recorded. It is not readily available in devices in which typed messages are spoken.

Written Output

Written output is also referred to as hard copy. It is the ability of the device to produce the message in print. Some communication devices have a built-in printer. These devices usually produce messages on small "strip" printers such as on a cash register slip. When a device does not have a built-in printer it may be equipped with a port for a small, portable printer. The portable printer may be set up at all times or connected only when needed. If the patient frequently leaves the house with the communication device, the addition of a portable printer may make the device somewhat cumbersome. If a larger printer is needed, the device is interfaced with a computer and the message can be printed on standard letter-size paper.

Software

Dedicated communication devices have the software already programmed into the device. Nondedicated communication devices have the software installed from a disk or CD ROM. Some software is equipped with only alphabet spelling, which allows the individual to generate any message desired. For those who are unable to read or write, special software programs are designed to satisfy their needs. These programs may be equipped with symbols. Some software programs are designed to help "speed up" the rate with which a patient types out a message. These are called "keystroke saving" options. Keystroke saving options may take the form of abbreviation-expansion or word prediction.

Abbreviation expansion allows the patient to store long words, phrases, or sentences in the device's memory using an alphabet code. Instead of spelling out a whole word, phrase, or sentence, the code is put in and the message is automatically retrieved (for example, HY = "Hello, how are you?"). *Word prediction* is a software option in which the communication device tries to "guess" or predict what the individual will say next. A list of possible word choices is presented to the patient. If the desired word is on the list, the individual only needs to select a number. If the choice is not on the list, the patient continues typing the word until the computer makes a correct prediction. Some software learns the patient's word usage over time and predicts words based on the individual's actual vocabulary.

Keyboard Emulation

Some electronic communication aids are designed to work with a personal computer by taking the place of the computer keyboard. This is known as *keyboard emulation.* The individual can run a personal computer (PC) by interfacing the PC and communication device. The PC will accept input regardless of the access method. However, the PC and the communication device must be compatible. Additionally, the patient will have to purchase an interface cable designed for that communication device and possibly a piece of hardware for the PC. Nondedicated communication devices do not have the keyboard emulation feature because they are already designed to accept all types of software.

Some communication devices claim transparency or compatibility with commercially available software programs (e.g., spreadsheet programs). Transparency means that the communication software is available and workable with nonspecialized programs, such as commercially available workplace software. Although many communication device manufacturers claim transparency, it is best to explore this feature with the specific programs that the patient plans to use.

Portability

Some communication devices are designed to be highly portable, with others designed to be mounted on a wheelchair or table top. Although portable devices may fit into a patient's lifestyle, they may have fewer features than less portable models. For example, a portable device may not have speech synthesis or a printer. When a speech synthesizer and printer are added, the device becomes heavier, more cumbersome, and less portable. The importance of speech and writing must be considered when selecting a highly portable system.

What is a "switch" and how is it used with electronic communication systems?

A switch is used to operate a communication device when the individual does not have the ability to use his or her fingers or hands. A switch is connected to the electronic communication device and acts as a kind of control unit. When activated by only one touch or movement, the switch sends a command to the communication device to start or stop. The device is controlled by a patient each time the switch is touched. There are many switches available today. Some are pictured in Figure 6. These switches are designed to meet the needs of individuals with differing degrees and types of physical weakness.

Switches may be activated with any part of the body, including the hand, foot, cheek, eyebrow, eyelid, and so on. A switch is chosen according to a patient's physical motor capabilities. However, because physical motor capability deteriorates with ALS/MND, the SLP must choose a switch that can meet the individual's anticipated changing abilities. Often, an infrared switch is selected. An infrared switch sends out a beam of light. When something passes quickly in front of this beam of light, the switch is activated. Therefore, an infrared switch does not have to be touched in order to send a signal. It is very sensitive and can accommodate those who have only minimal movements.

I have heard that a switch can be used in many ways. What are some of the different ways?

A switch can also be combined with a buzzer to form an alerting signal. This is a pre-established signal designed to get someone's attention or call for help in an emergency. This is especially important for an individual who has little or no speech and cannot call out for help. The most important factor in choosing an alerting signal is an awareness of the individual's physical motor limitations. The individual must be able to activate the switch/buzzer combination at any time.

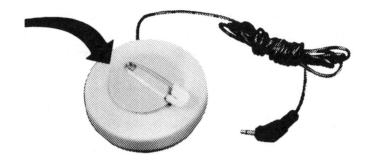

a

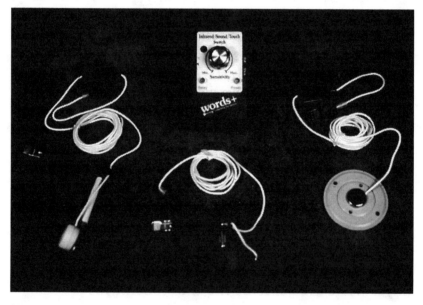

b

Figure 6. a. A pillow switch (Photo courtesy of Crestwood Company). **b.** An infra-red switch (Photo courtesy of Words Plus)

Alerting systems are an important consideration for hospitalized individuals. The SLP cannot assume that the patient will be able to activate the standard nursing call buzzer that is typically provided for hospital patients. A patient without the use of his or her hands may not be able to apply the pressure needed to "ring-in" and call a nurse for help. Therefore, customized switches must be available so that ALS/MND patients have access to nursing care at all times. The individual should speak to the SLP about acquiring a switch/buzzer alerting signal, even before such a setup is required.

A switch can also be used to activate an Environmental Control Unit (ECU). This is a system that allows the patient to control various home appliances, such as appliance on/off switches, television channels, or any other important electronic devices. An occupational therapist can assist in the selection of the correct ECU.

There are so many devices, how do I select the system that is best for me?

After the evaluation is complete the patient should understand the features offered by various electronic communication devices. It is essential that a SLP is used to assist in the selection of the most appropriate electronic communication device.

The selection of a communication device is highly individual and based on the communication lifestyle of the patient. There is tremendous variability in the communication needs of individuals. For example, if there are young children in the home who cannot read, it is essential that the communication device have the ability to speak. For those who want to continue to be employed, compatible software other than communication software may be needed. If the patient leads an active lifestyle that includes travel, a portable device will be essential.

The SLP assesses the communication needs of each individual by making a thorough evaluation of both the places in which the communication is going to occur and the partners with whom the communication will take place. Then, the SLP and the patient can consider the features offered by the various communication devices and select a device that best matches those needs and situations. The native language of the patient, visual/hearing abilities, and especially physical motor capability must be considered.

One of the most important considerations in selecting an electronic communication device is its methods of access. It must be remembered that ALS/MND is a progressive disease and it is essential that the selected device satisfies today's needs and anticipates future demands. The patient should choose a device that offers scanning as one of the available access methods. A device that allows scanning will permit even the most disabled patient to activate the device.

Unless one has no financial considerations, it is not wise to select a device with only direct selection access. Although the individual may be able to use the device at the time of the evaluation, he or she may not be able to use it in the future, and selection would be a costly error for those with limited financial resources. Many electronic communication aids permit a wide variety of access methods, including direct selection, Morse code, and scanning. The access methods on the selected communication device must accommodate the potential continued physical motor deterioration. The SLP who specializes in augmentative communication will determine the best system to meet the patient's ongoing needs.

What can I do to help my speech-language pathologist select a system that is right for me?

Patients should spend some time thinking about all of their different communication environments, partners, and needs. The "Communication Needs Assessment" (see Appendix A) is designed to help patients consolidate the necessary information for the speech-language pathologist. The more the patient understands and communicates his or her needs to the speech-language pathologist, the more effective the speech-language pathologist can be in determining which communication systems will be most appropriate. The speech-language pathologist will develop ways to meet each patient's needs, despite physical limitations.

Now that I have my communication system, does it mean that I should stop talking?

A well-designed communication system allows the patient to use all of his or her available communicative resources. That means that a patient who can still talk may combine speech with writing or pointing on an alphabet board. An individual who can still write may use pencil and paper when going to the grocery store, but use a computer at home for sending lengthy messages. In a successful communication system, communication skills are maintained until they are no longer viable.

A well-designed communication system allows the patient to spontaneously generate any message he or she desires. This is best done by giving the patient access to the alphabet. Pictures or symbols are not necessary unless the patient using the system cannot read or write, or must communicate with an individual who speaks another language. However, the alphabet may be combined with picture communication if that better meets the patient's needs.

Now that I have my communication device, who will teach me to use it?

The SLP has not fully completed the job once the communication system is selected. The SLP is also responsible for teaching the patient how to use the electronic communication device and how to integrate all the available methods of communication into his or her life.

Additionally, because of the progressive nature of ALS/MND, the SLP must prepare the individual to use methods of communication that are designed to work with deteriorating physical motor skills. The SLP must anticipate any potential changes in the patient's condition, so that he or she is never without a usable means of communication.

Are there ways for me to communicate by telephone?

The SLP should always consider phone use when designing a communication system. Those who have understandable speech may consider a speaker phone for hands-free operation. If speech becomes too difficult to understand by phone, an alternative should be considered. For an individual who can still type, a TDD (Telecommunication Device for the Deaf) may be appropriate. The patient types the phone message into the TDD. The message is then transmitted to a listener who has a TDD unit in the home or office. If the listener does not have a TDD unit, the message is read to the listener by the operator via a service called the Relay Center. This service is available through the telephone company. A TDD is very useful for patients who can still write messages during face-to-face communication, but need assistance with phone usage. All messages are kept confidential by Relay Centers.

Patients with ALS/MND who do not have the ability to type may use an electronic communication device with synthesized speech to talk over the phone. Additionally, the patient may consider purchase of telephone software for a personal or laptop computer. This software dials the phone and then converts a typed message into speech that can be heard by the listener.

Is there a way for me to use my electronic communication system to communicate with other patients?

Communication with individuals who are not in the same location is possible over the phone lines through a computer and a modem. A modem allows a nonspeaking person to use the phone by typing messages and communicating in writing to other people who have similar systems. An on-line service (e.g., CompuServe, America On-Line, Prodigy) is selected and the individual has access to a group of people who make up discussion groups, forums, and so on. Through an on-line service, people can leave messages for each other and retrieve them for later use. This is called electronic mail (e-mail). It is the computer equivalent of postal mail.

Messages are sent using an individual's electronic address. These addresses have a format that varies depending on the on-line service that is being used by the individual. Patients can communicate with each other from different parts of the world when they have a computer, a modem and are connected to an on-line service. On-line services have a monthly charge which is billed to the user.

I'm told that electronic communication systems are expensive. How can I get help to pay for it?

The term "funding" refers to the means by which individuals pay for needed equipment, such as an electronic communication device and, sometimes, for the services of the SLP. Private insurance companies have been known to fund communication devices because they are considered "durable medical equipment" and prosthetic devices that are necessary to dictate medical needs and participate in one's own medical care. Medicare and approximately a dozen Medicaid programs consider AAC devices as prosthetics. Medicare has traditionally not funded communication devices, but Medicare has approved funding for at least one device, a computer-based system, following an administrative appeal. Over the past few years, Medicaid has become more aware of the role of communication in patient care and more willing to fund electronic communication devices. However, the SLP must adhere to strict guidelines when evaluating and requesting the equipment.

Some private organizations have shown a willingness to fund communication devices, including churches, synagogues, fraternal organizations, and businesses. Often families of ALS/MND patients are willing to donate equipment when it is no longer needed. There are a number of published references that can help SLPs and families identify potential funding sources for a patient. Some examples are given in Appendix C. The speech-language pathologist takes an active role in justifying the need for equipment for appropriate candidates.

My doctor tells me that I have to have a tracheotomy to help me breathe and manage my secretions. Is this going to interfere with my speech and swallowing? What exactly is a tracheostomy tube? What is a ventilator? Can I live at home with these?

Some patients may develop difficulty using their respiratory muscles to breathe and cough. Mechanical devices can assist a patient with this problem. Noninvasive mechanical ventilation is the use of a machine (ventilator), which gives breaths through a mask, mouthpiece, or small nosepiece. The individual wears the device at specific times of the day to support breathing. In addition, a machine called an exsufflator can actually mimic a cough by puffing air into the throat, then pulling it out via suction or reverse pressure. This is not painful. It actually helps to pull out secretions from the lungs that cannot be cleared by a weak cough, and, therefore, assists in keeping the lungs healthy.

Eventually, some patients may require a tracheostomy. A tracheotomy is the surgical creation of an opening in the trachea, or windpipe. A tracheostomy tube is a plastic or metal tube that fits into that hole to keep it open, allowing instruments such as suction catheters to be inserted. Respirators or ventilators can be attached to the tube. Tracheotomies are performed when a patient needs assistance breathing and cannot receive it by less invasive means (such as a mask over the mouth or nose). Usually this occurs because secretions have become too difficult to manage—that is, to remove by coughing. Secretions then block the throat or airway and must be manually removed through the tube. This process is not painful, but care must be taken to keep the tracheostomy area clean. This need for sterile technique and the possible need for the respirator or ventilator (the machine that gives mechanical breaths) requires special care in the home. This may mean careful training for family members, the presence of a nurse, and periodic visits by a respiratory therapist. Many people live at home successfully with tracheostomies and ventilators. Services are available from specialized home care agencies.

At times, the presence of the tracheostomy tube can interfere with speech and swallowing. The speech-language pathologist and respiratory therapist can work with the physician to make adjustments, such as using special tracheostomy tubes or attachments (i.e., one-way speaking valves) to allow speech and facilitate safe swallowing. These special tubes or speaking valves allow patients to produce a spoken voice even when tracheostomy tubes and ventilators are necessary. One-way speaking valves are especially useful, as patients need not put their finger on the tube to speak. Air is directed into the tracheostomy tube during inhalation and then instead of exiting back out of the tube during exhalation, the air is directed upward to reach the vocal folds to allow speech/voice production. This is why it is referred to as a one-way valve. Air goes in but cannot go back out the way it entered. As with all issues of communication and swallowing, a careful and individual assessment is required.

In some cases, speech is not possible, even with using special tracheostomy tubes or speaking valves. When verbal communication is no longer possible, alternative or augmentative communication methods may be necessary.

Swallowing Intervention

This section is divided into a series of questions to assist you in understanding how to address swallowing problems in ALS/MND.

What is dysphagia (swallowing impairment)?

Dysphagia is a disruption of the normal swallowing process. Dysphagia may lead to an inability to eat and drink adequate amounts or an inability to swallow safely. Dysphagia is caused by the progressive muscular weakness that occurs with ALS/MND. Most patients will experience some changes in the ability to take food and liquid by mouth (orally) during the disease process. Dysphagia can be a life-threatening condition for several reasons. Patients and caregivers must be aware of early signs and symptoms so that compensatory strategies can be immediately provided to address the problems.

When the dysphagia is severe, oral intake of foods or liquids may be inadequate, with resulting weight loss or dehydration. One consequence of dysphagia can be aspiration pneumonia, an infection caused by entry of a foreign material, such as saliva, food, or liquid, into the lungs. This material breeds bacteria, which then leads to the pneumonia. If large enough amounts of any material enter the airway or passage leading to the lungs, choking may occur. These consequences of dysphagia are quite severe.

Therefore it is important to recognize the signs and symptoms of a swallowing disorder before these more severe difficulties occur. As with other aspects of ALS/MND, the approach to dysphagia should be proactive. In other words, early identification of symptoms is important in the management of swallowing problems and assists the medical team in facilitating safe swallowing strategies. This can avoid life-threatening problems and often extends the amount of time an individual can continue to eat by mouth safely and with enjoyment.

How do we swallow normally?

To deal with dysphagia, it is important to understand the basics of the swallowing process. The normal swallowing process is illustrated in Figure 7. We take swallowing for granted and do not realize that it is a complex series of events that happens in different stages. ALS/MND affects each of the stages and so can create multiple problems.

The first stage of swallowing is called the oral stage. This is when food or liquid is first introduced into the mouth. At this point we often refer to the food or liquid as the bolus. A bolus is simply a mass. The bolus is chewed, if necessary, and then moved quickly (1–2 seconds) from the front to the back of the mouth. The lips, tongue, and jaw are active during this process. The tongue is especially important in controlling and moving the bolus in the mouth and for placing the bolus at the back of the mouth in readiness for the next phase of swallowing—the pharyngeal phase.

The pharynx is another name for the part of the throat through which the bolus moves, so the *pharyngeal phase* refers to the time the bolus leaves the mouth and moves into the throat. A very important part of the swallow process happens at this point. It is here that what we think of as the actual swallow occurs. This is a response by nerves and muscles triggered by the brain. Several things happen. The muscles in the pharynx contract and start to push the food down. At the same time, the entrance to the windpipe, or larynx, closes and rises. This is a vital time, because as the food goes down the pharynx, it passes directly over the larynx. This is when the vocal cords close, protecting the lungs from any liquid or food.

Although the pharynx leads to the esophagus and stomach, the larynx leads to the windpipe and lungs. The larynx normally protects itself by rising via muscle action, moving out of the way of the bolus, and closing the vocal folds. After the bolus passes over and moves down the

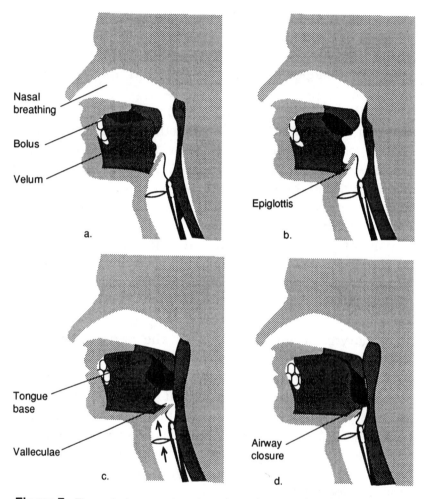

Figure 7. The oral, pharyngeal, and esophageal stages of swallowing. The bolus is propelled in a posterior direction **(a)** as the tongue base retracts and the velum elevates **(b–c)**. The larynx begins to elevate **(c–d)** as the bolus descends into the pharynx. As the bolus passes through the upper esophageal sphincter

pharynx, the larynx descends and resumes its usual position. This entire process only takes a second or two. The bolus continues to the third phase of the swallow, the esophageal phase.

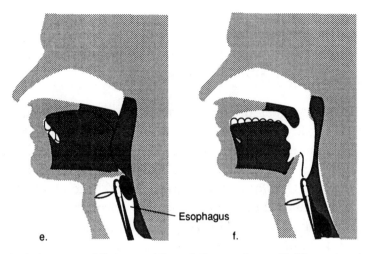

Esophagus

e.   f.

(e), the bolus moves fully into and through the esophagus (f). The oral and pharyngeal phases last approximately 1 second each. The esophageal phase varies between approximately 8 to 20 seconds.

The esophagus is the tube of muscle that leads to the stomach. As the bolus leaves the pharynx, the top of the esophagus begins to relax so that the bolus can enter. Once the bolus is in the esophagus, muscles push it through to the stomach. This phase of swallowing is usually the longest.

The stages of the swallow are under both voluntary and involuntary control. This means that certain aspects of the swallow can be modified more than others. The oral and pharyngeal phases have mixed voluntary and involuntary control, although the esophageal is entirely involuntary.

How can ALS/MND affect the normal swallowing process?

As ALS/MND can affect the lips, tongue, and jaw muscles, the oral phase of the swallow can be affected. Problems occur with keeping the lips closed, opening and closing the mouth, and moving the bolus in the mouth. Drooling, inability to close the lips on a straw or spoon, and reduced chewing ability may result.

In the pharyngeal phase, the muscles of the throat may become weak. There is often decreased ability to "trigger," or start, the actual swallow. Problems closing the vocal cords also occur during this stage. This results in food sticking in the pharynx. Coughing or choking is noted as food drops into the larynx instead of moving normally through the pharynx into the stomach. It is in this stage that aspiration, or entry of food or liquid into the windpipe, usually occurs.

ALS/MND can also affect the muscle tone of the esophagus. This causes food to sit in the esophagus without moving, or perhaps return back up from the stomach (reflux). Patients often refer to this sensation as heartburn.

How is dysphagia managed?

The first step in dealing with dysphagia is a careful evaluation to pinpoint the stage at which problems occur. The team members who are vital in this process are the speech-language pathologist, physician, dietitian, and occupational therapist.

What is the role of the speech-language pathologist during the dysphagia evaluation process?

The speech-language pathologist (SLP) often begins the swallowing evaluation by observing the patient at mealtime. The individual may be asked to eat foods and liquids that are generally the most difficult for most people. The clinician notes the symptoms that occur. Some of the possible observations might include drooling or coughing on specific foods or liquids. Although this important initial step can give the clinician an idea of what stages of swallowing are impaired, the process cannot stop at this point. Only some of the problems involving the oral stage of swallowing can actually be observed. Special, objective tests for all stages are needed to document dysfunction. The speech-language pathologist, working with various physicians, will participate in these assessments.

What objective tests are used in the assessment of dysphagia?

The first of these tests, performed by the otolaryngologist (ENT) with the speech-language pathologist (SLP) is a direct visualization of the throat or pharynx during swallowing called a *fiberoptic swallowing study.* The ENT inserts a special instrument, a thin, flexible scope with a tiny camera on the end, into the patient's nose and through to the throat. The ENT and SLP can look at the status of many structures of the throat, including the vocal folds, at the beginning of the fiberoptic study. Then, food or liquid (usually colored with vegetable dye) is given. As the food passes through the pharynx, it is possible to see if it becomes stuck at any place, or if it enters the larynx (windpipe).

The fiberoptic study is very helpful, but only one evaluation can assess the entire swallowing process and follow the food entering the mouth and into the stomach (the oral to the esophageal stage). This is an X-ray test known by several names, including a *modified barium swallow* or *videofluoroscopy.* It is sometimes confused with an esophagram.

A *barium swallow* or *esophagram* does what the name implies—studies the esophageal phase of swallowing. This leaves out two vital stages! Patients need a test that can evaluate all three stages of swallowing. During a *videofluoroscopy*, the radiologist and the speech-language pathologist work together. The patient swallows carefully measured amounts of different types of food and liquid. The speech-language pathologist records the patient's response to each type of food and notes where problems occur. The videofluoroscopy can be used to evaluate different trial therapy techniques. The X-ray study is captured on videotape. The patient will see the bolus of food which can be seen as darker material actually move from the mouth into the throat and then into the esophagus. Specific problem areas and recommendations for therapy can be discussed as the speech-language pathologist and patient view the videotape together after the evaluation has been completed.

I don't have any trouble eating food or drinking liquid, but I am having difficulty with my saliva, especially at night. What can I do about it?

There are different medications that can be tried to decrease excess saliva. Unfortunately, many individuals report only limited success. These medications can also have undesirable side effects. Patients should discuss medication options with their doctor. It is very important for the patient to try to keep hydrated (ingest ample liquids), which helps keep the saliva from becoming too thick and unmanageable. Papaya juice is a helpful liquid that contains a substance that reduces the thickness of the saliva.

Your SLP or doctor may recommend that you elevate the head of your bed at night to reduce pooling of saliva in the throat. If saliva becomes excessive, a portable suction machine can be used to gently and effectively remove it from the mouth.

What type of therapy can be offered to a patient with a swallowing problem?

The videofluoroscopic study is usually the first place that the SLP can tell which therapy will help a person with a swallowing disorder. Therapy can be thought of in two ways: trying to improve an underlying weakness or compensating for a problem that exists.

Muscle exercises can address problems in the oral and pharyngeal phases. For example, if the SLP sees that the tongue cannot push the food through the mouth, the patient can practice strengthening exercises for the tongue by pushing against a tongue stick or metal spoon. Lip exercises and being aware of lip position during swallowing can help control drooling. Special exercises that make the larynx move up and down, such as pitch exercises, may strengthen weak throat muscles.

The speech-language pathologist can also teach the patient compensatory strategies to deal with a specific problem. For example, a patient may cough and choke while drinking liquids, with videofluoroscopy confirming this symptom and showing that aspiration is taking place. To prevent liquid from entering the larynx, the SLP may try to teach the individual to consciously hold his or her breath before swallowing. This can reduce the risk of aspiration. Whether the patient can learn this technique may depend on the stage of his or her disease, but it can be very effective in preventing aspiration (the entrance of food or liquid into the lungs) by targeting and strengthening weakened throat muscles. Aspiration of food or liquid puts an individual at risk for developing aspiration pneumonia. This can be life-threatening and very dangerous for an individual with ALS/MND.

Strategies to help compensate for weak aspects of a swallow are very helpful. These are often referred to as postural modifications because they involve changing the positions in which people eat. For example, turning the head so food will not go down the weak side of the throat is one strategy. Of course, it is important for the SLP to know that these postural changes work by trying them out during the videofluoroscopy to actually see what happens with and without each strategy.

The way that a patient eats is an area that can be addressed in treatment. The rate of eating and amount of food that is placed in the mouth at one time is carefully assessed, often during the first mealtime observation by the therapist. It may not be possible for the individual to eat as quickly or as much as before the disease. Chewing, for example, can quickly tire someone whose muscles are weak. Therefore, the therapist may ask the patient to eat slowly, taking small amounts of food in each bite.

As it may be hard to take in adequate nutrition eating this way, smaller meals at more frequent intervals may be suggested. The person with ALS/MND may eat six small meals a day instead of three large ones. Frequent snacks can also be a good idea. The registered dietitian is a good person to consult when arranging these "mini-meals" and snacks. Although the way that the patient eats is important, the type of food taken is also vital to the patient with dysphagia. Dietary modifications are one way to eat safely and well as long as possible.

What kind of changes in my diet may be necessary?

At each stage of the disease, the individual with dysphagia may need diet modifications to meet changing abilities. As the muscles change and become weak, one of the first modifications may be moving from regular foods that must be chewed to softer consistencies that require less chewing. From this point, chopped food and then eventually pureed consistencies may be needed. Pureed boluses are often easier to manage, because they stay together in the mouth and throat, even when it takes a long time to swallow. They are usually less likely to stick in the throat. Dietary changes are an individual process; they should be guided by an SLP who can assess what types of food are best tolerated at a given point in the disease. Hints on food preparation are also provided. Pureed food does not mean "baby food!" Just about any type of food can be put through a food processor and then prepared in a way that is pleasant to the palate and the eye. This may mean putting a pureed carrot back into its regular shape even after it has gone through its consistency changes (to look like a carrot again).

The most important change in consistency to be aware of is the use of thickening agents for liquids. Liquids are often hard to tolerate because they move through the mouth and throat so quickly. They are hard to control, in contrast to something thicker, like pudding, that stays together. But liquids are vital in avoiding dehydration. The SLP may thus suggest that the patient use a powder in liquid which thickens it to varying degrees. This tasteless powder can allow a patient to continue safely taking liquids long past the point where a regular, "thin" liquid might be aspirated. Videofluoroscopy is again used to document the need for a thickener.

If I can no longer eat by mouth, what are my options?

If the disease progresses to the point that food cannot be taken orally, the patient may be asked to consider an alternate form of taking nutrition, usually a tube into the stomach through which a liquid supplement is given. This is most often called a gastrostomy tube or percutaneous gastrostomy tube (PEG). A gastrostomy tube does not effect a person's ability to swallow in any way. It merely provides an additional or alternative means of getting nutrition and hydration despite a severe swallowing impairment.

Many patients accept a tube while they are still eating to assist in taking in adequate amounts of nutrition and hydration. As with other decisions, such as accepting a ventilator, acceptance of a tube can be a difficult decision, and is very individualized.

How does the physician put the tube in my stomach?

The procedure for a PEG can be performed in an outpatient setting. General anesthesia is usually not necessary for placement of this tube. A local anesthetic is used to numb the area where the incision is made in the stomach. Other types of tubes may require a slightly more complicated surgical procedure. Your doctor should explain all the options to you.

The ALS/MND Team

This section describes the professionals who may be involved in helping patients with ALS/MDD meet their ongoing needs and optimize their lifestyles.

Who are the professionals who assist the patient with communication and swallowing needs?

It is crucial to the patient's overall management to have a coordinated care program. When team members work together in a multidisciplinary fashion, they can set up mutually agreed upon goals to optimize quality of life.

Patient and Caregiver

The patient and caregiver are an integral part of the ALS/MND team. As the patient obtains information assisting him or her to become an educated consumer, he or she can make more educated decisions. The team must always include the patient, as he or she ultimately has the authority to make the final decision in all aspects of care.

Physicians

The primary care physician is responsible for the overall medical management of a patient, including the prescription of medications, timing of special tests or treatments, and referrals to other specialists. The primary care physician is often an internist or general family practitioner (GP) who is often familiar with the patient's medical history prior to the onset of the disease. The internist or GP will make referrals to other physicians who specialize in the diagnosis and treatment of respiratory and neurological conditions.

These may include a neurologist, who is usually responsible for the initial diagnosis and periodic follow-up of the neurological condition; a pulmonologist, who is often called on when respiratory problems develop; an otolaryngologist, who assesses the status of the airway (vocal cords); a physiatrist, who assesses and assists in the rehabilitation of the patient; and a gastroenterologist, who is responsible for determining candidacy for alternate forms of feeding and for the surgical placement of a feeding tube or gastrostomy. Other medical specialists may also be called upon during various stages of the disease to assist in the overall management of the disease process.

Speech-Language Pathologist

The speech-language pathologist (SLP) is responsible for assessing and treating the communication and swallowing needs of a patient with ALS/MND. It is the role of the SLP to ensure that the patient can communicate during each stage of the disease process. Communication methods involve both oral and nonoral approaches. Oral communication approaches may include verbal communication supplemented with writing or use of an alphabet board when there is a breakdown with traditional communication. For those who use a ventilator to help with breathing, the SLP, working closely with the respiratory therapist, may manipulate the tracheostomy tube or ventilator to allow the patient to produce voice and communicate verbally. The SLP focuses on maintaining muscle strength for as long a period as possible, while monitoring functional communication status and ensuring that a patient is able to transfer needed messages throughout a day.

If oral communication becomes nonfunctional, the SLP intervenes with alternative or augmentative communication systems. These systems can either supplement oral/verbal communication or replace speech. The SLP works closely with other team members, such as the occupational therapist and rehabilitation engineer, to ensure that an individual can access and utilize a chosen communication system in a variety of settings.

The maintenance of safe swallowing is another area of focus for the SLP. Swallowing impairment often occurs when there is deterioration in oral muscle strength. The SLP provides a comprehensive assessment and treatment approach to swallowing disorders and attempts to maintain the patient on oral feedings for as long as possible. Diet modification and compensatory strategies are part of the SLP's treatment philosophy.

Rehabilitation Engineer

The expertise of rehabilitation engineers varies from individual to individual. The rehabilitation engineer who best meets the needs of the ALS/MND population is one who is familiar with augmentative communication systems (ACS), switch access strategies, environmental control units, and the mounting of either or both to a wheelchair.

The rehabilitation engineer is a resource person to be utilized in conjunction with other health care professionals, such as SLPs or occupational therapists. He or she may assist in making an appropriate selection of a sophisticated switch or device. Users of technology can benefit from the viewpoint of rehabilitation engineers, as they provide information on technology safety, operation, maintenance, mounting, and operating precautions.

Technical problems that arise can be resolved quickly by an individual with a technical background such as rehabilitation engineer. It is useful for the rehabilitation engineer to have a knowledge of personal computers.

Rehabilitation engineers often keep current on the latest technological advances in technology. He or she can sift through the technical jargon manufacturers may use to sell their products. Patients should be able to ask the rehabilitation engineer whether a product being considered for purchase is compatible with products already in use. If the product is not compatible, questions such as "can it be upgraded?" may be asked by the patient.

Social Worker

The social worker can provide the ongoing support and counseling that a patient with a degenerative condition requires. Through counseling sessions, the social worker can address the issues of quality of life and facilitate problem solving as the patient experiences changes during the course of the disease.

The social worker focuses on the psychosocial needs of the patient, as well as assisting in financial planning, helping to establish a network of referral sources and support groups, and facilitates transfer to extended care facilities, if necessary. The social worker is an advocate for the patient and assists the patient in the decision-making process by providing ongoing education on multiple issues. The social worker can provide information on surrogate decision making, living wills, and laws in the state in which the patient lives. Families and patients can rely on the social worker to explain the intricacies of private and federal insurance programs and to help in coping with possible loss of income that may accompany long-term disability.

The social worker will work closely with the augmentative communication team if funding for an electronic communication system occurs. The social worker may facilitate contacts with private insurers and provide information necessary in making the funding process more successful.

Psychologist

An individual with a chronic disease such as ALS/MND will experience many different adjustment problems and will have a variety of emotional reactions. The most immediate psychological difficulties are affected by the duration of the disease and/or disability, as well as the level of physical challenge. The psychologist is trained to work with people experiencing anxiety, depression, and anger, reactions which may weaken an individual's and family's motivation and general well-being.

Adjustment to ALS/MND will require coping with radical changes in lifestyle, self-image, and interpersonal relationships. The effective psychologist is also sensitive to how a change in communication will further challenge an individual and should be capable of responding positively to stated and unstated needs. Any psychologist working with a patient with ALS/MND or the family must be aware of the communicative needs of the individual and the range of challenges presented to caregivers. Many therapeutic interventions (individual psychotherapy, short-term focused groups, psychosocial support, stress management, assertiveness, and life-planning/bereavement intervention) may be useful at different times.

Occupational Therapist

The occupational therapist's (OT) primary role is to assess and provide intervention to maximize a patient's activities of daily living. These activities include dressing, feeding, washing, and any other daily routines normally followed.

Assessment of fine motor control is integral to the OT's assessment, as recommendations in facilitating daily activities may be enhanced by use of adaptive devices.

These devices allow a patient to independently continue performing tasks. Facilitating increased independence is demonstrated by the use of environmental controls.

The OT may be responsible for providing devices that allow the patient to manipulate the environment when physical disability interferes with independent control. For example, the use of an environmental control unit allows a patient who is quadriplegic to turn lights on and off, make telephone calls, or control a radio or television. The OT works closely with the SLP and rehabilitation engineer, as an augmentative communication system may incorporate environmental options that need to be adapted to the needs of an individual.

The occupational therapist is a valuable member of the augmentative communication team. Positioning for optimal seating in a wheelchair, as well as selection and positioning of a switch, is incorporated in the OT's treatment program.

Dietitian

The dietitian, or nutritionist, assesses nutritional status whether feeding is oral or nonoral (feeding via a gastrostomy tube). With the assistance of laboratory blood analysis, the dietician can objectively monitor a patient's nutritional status. The dietitian is also skilled in the subjective analysis of overall physical status (e.g., skin appearance) as an indicator of possible nutritional deficiencies. Recommendations can be made for dietary supplements, such as high-calorie, high-protein drinks and foods that will provide the additional calories and vitamins and minerals needed to maintain weight.

The dietitian works closely with the SLP to recommend a diet that is best managed by the patient. Consistencies can be easily modified to allow for safe swallowing and that also ensure adequate nutrition and liquids. If swallowing problems increase, the dietitian will work closely with the patient to recommend formulas to be taken via a gastrostomy tube. Altering formula type can easily be prescribed by the dietitian if tolerance of milk-based products is a problem or if fiber needs to be added to assist in bowel movements.

Respiratory Therapist

The respiratory therapist's (RT) role is to monitor the patient's medical and respiratory status with special monitoring devices. The RT works with the physician to carefully monitor a patient's respiratory status to ensure that adequate oxygenation is maintained. If the patient is on a ventilator, the RT is responsible for maintaining and setting up the mechanical ventilator. The RT often teaches the patient and caregiver about the specific ventilatory device employed and ensures that controls are set to the specifications of the physician.

The RT works closely with the speech-language pathologist when modifications to the ventilator are necessary to facilitate speech. The professionals work together to maintain adequate ventilatory support while attempting to allow for speech for as long as possible. The RT also assists in making necessary changes to the tracheostomy tube and ventilator to facilitate safe swallowing.

Physical Therapist

The physical therapist's (PT) role extends beyond traditional therapy when working with the patient with ALS/MND. Assessment focuses on muscle function of the arms and legs, as well as evaluation of the respiratory musculature. Treatment during the initial stages of the disease involves muscle strengthening and movement exercises designed to maintain the patient's mobility for as long as possible. The PT's role is to instruct the patient as well as the caregiver in proper techniques to move and exercise the arms and legs. These are referred to as active or passive range of motion exercises.

For bed-bound patients, the PT in conjunction with the occupational therapist assesses bed positioning needs and evaluates the patient's potential for contractures. Devices to improve comfort and ensure best positioning in bed for patient use of an augmentative communication system may be provided.

The PT may also provide a specialized service by offering chest physical therapy. This includes evaluation of chest wall mobility for the clearance of secretions as well as postural drainage or placing the patient in various positions to mobilize the secretions in the chest. Along with instruction on how to produce as productive a cough as possible, the PT may work with the patient to facilitate movement of mucus that accumulates in the chest. This may be difficult for a patient because of weakened respiratory musculature.

Glossary

abbreviation expansion = A keystroke-saving feature offered by many computer communication software programs. This feature allows users to type two or three letters to abbreviate short phrases or sentences. When the patient puts in these letters, an entire phrase or sentence can be spoken or written.

airway = Entrance into the lungs.

alerting signal/buzzer = A means of calling attention to begin a conversation or for an emergency situation. The buzzer is connected to a switch that the patient activates within the individual's physical ability. A loud sound is produced when the switch is activated.

anarthria = A condition in which the patient can no longer produce any speech or sound to communicate. It may happen in the late stages of ALS/MND.

aspiration pneumonia = A lung infection caused by foreign material entering the trachea (windpipe) and passing into the lungs. This foreign material may be food, liquid, or saliva that can no longer be safely swallowed by the patient.

augmentative and alternative communication system (AAC) = A method of communication that utilizes one or a combination of many forms of message transmission, including speech, sign, gesture, writing, alphabet boards, word charts, and so on. Some AAC systems incorporate the use of electronic components such as computers, speech synthesizers, and printers. The patient is using an *augmentative system* when speech is combined with other forms of communication. The patient is using an *alternative system* when speech has been completely replaced by other forms of communication.

dedicated electronic communication devices = An electronic communication system that has been developed solely for the purpose of communication.

digitized speech = Artificial speech that has been compiled from recordings of human speech. Digitized speech has excellent intelligibility. Some electronic communication systems have digitized speech as an option.

direct selection = A method of choosing a language item from a communication system by pointing with a part of the body such as the hand, head, eyes, etc. This method may be used with both nonelectronic and electronic communication systems.

dysarthria = A condition in which the muscles for speech are weakened, thereby affecting the intelligibility of speech. The resulting speech impairment may range from mild to severe.

dysphagia = A swallowing impairment resulting from weakening of the structures for swallowing including the lips, tongue, larynx (voice box), and pharynx (throat).

electronic mail (e-mail) = The computer equivalent of postal mail. Messages are composed with a word processor or specialized software. Messages are then addressed to another individual using their unique e-mail address. These addresses have a format that varies depending on the service you used (eg., 73523,151 is a CompuServe-style address, and 73523,151@CompuServe.com is an Internet style address). *See listing for* **modem**. When you are connected through a computer modem to your service, you are "on line."

esophageal phase = The third phase of the swallow. This phase begins as food leaves the pharynx and enters the esophagus.

esophagus = A muscular tube that allows the passage of food from the pharynx to the stomach. The peristaltic action of the esophagus (movement of the food downward) may deteriorate with the progression of ALS/MND.

exsufflator = A device that alternately delivers air and then suction to the airway to assist in removing secretions, phlegm or food from the lungs.

eyegaze = A method of selecting letters or words by looking at a desired item. Eyegaze may be used as a means of selecting from a nonelectronic system such as an Eye-Link or E-Tran. There are electronic eyegaze systems, but these may not be readily accessible for patients with ALS/MND.

fiberoptic swallowing study = A swallowing study that is conducted by passing a fiberoptic scope through the nose and above the vocal folds. The scope allows the structures involved in swallowing to be seen. After food has been given at the beginning of the study, the doctor and speech-language pathologist can see if any food remains in the area of the vocal folds, or has entered the airway.

hard copy = The term for written output of a communication system.

infrared switch = A switch that works by emitting a beam of light. When something passes through the beam, the switch is activated. This switch is widely used by patients with ALS/MND because it does not have to be touched. Its only requirement is that the patient have movement of a small body part (usually the eye or eyelid).

Internet = An immense interconnection of computers that share a common transmission method. Users take part by sending electronic mail to other users at their Internet address. Specialized technical knowledge is not necessary.

keyboard emulation = A function of dedicated electronic communication systems in which a separate personal or laptop computer can be operated through the communication device. Through the use of an interfacing cable and specialized hardware, the communication device takes the place of the computer keyboard. Information can also be transferred from the device and stored in the computer.

larynx = The structure that connects the mouth and pharynx (throat) with the trachea (windpipe). The larynx, also called the voice box, houses the vocal folds. It is the passage of air through these folds that give a person the ability to produce a voice. The vocal folds are also an important structure in swallowing. The larynx rises up and the vocal folds close when swallowing occurs so that food does not enter the trachea (windpipe).

modem = A device that is internally or externally connected to a personal computer that allows one computer to "talk" to another over normal phone lines. It works with telecommunication software.

modified barium swallow = An X-ray examination in which food may be tracked as it passes from the mouth to the esophagus. This examination provides objective information about a patient's ability to swallow food safely. It may also provide information about the best types of food for the patient with ALS/MND to be eating (also called a **videofluoroscopy**).

on-line = When your computer is connected via a modem to another computer, bulletin board system or on-line service.

on-line service = An electronic community that is composed of forums, discussion, groups, meeting area, electronic mail, file libraries. Through a service, people connect their computers to other computers through telephone lines to exchange ideas, conversation, interests, and so on. You can do anything from a search of an encyclopedia to go shopping in an electronic mall. The more popular services like CompuServe and Prodigy charge a small monthly fee (typically $8 to $14). This includes access to a variety of basic services.

oral stage = The first stage of swallowing. Food enters the mouth, is chewed, and is moved to the back of the mouth, ready to be swallowed.

pharyngeal phase = This swallowing stage begins when the swallow is triggered. Food moves through the pharynx until it gets to the esophagus.

pharynx = A muscular tube that forms the throat. It connects the nose and mouth to both the esophagus (food pipe) and trachea (windpipe). The pharynx is important for both breathing and eating.

scanning = A method of accessing a communication system in which the message units (letters, pictures) are presented to the patient with ALS/MND in groups. The patient with ALS/MND waits until the desired item is shown and then chooses it. Scanning may be used as an access method with both nonelectronic and electronic communication systems.

synthesized speech = Artificial speech that has been formulated by electronically combining sounds to obtain a human quality. Synthesized speech ranges in intelligibility from poor to excellent.

telecommunication software = A program that allows control of a modem connected to a computer to call another computer. These programs help automate the tasks of dialing and entering your name and password.

tracheotomy = A surgical procedure/creation that creates an opening into the trachea or windpipe. Once the opening has been created, a tracheostomy tube is placed to keep it safely open.

transparency = This term is used to mean that the special functions offered by the communication software (i.e., single-finger access, mouse emulation) are also available when the patient is using non-specialized software, such as spreadsheet or database software.

videofluoroscopy = A radiological procedure performed jointly by radiology and speech pathology departments. This examination specifically evaluates the oral, pharyngeal, and esophageal phases of swallowing (also referred to as a modified barium swallow).

word prediction = A keystroke saving option offered by some communication software manufacturers that allows the system to "guess" what the patient is typing. While typing an entry, the computer offers possible choices of words that the patient may want to use. If the desired word is on the list, the patient selects a number and the word appears. The computer then attempts to guess the following word. The patient saves keystrokes by being able to choose a single number instead of spelling an entire word.

APPENDIX A

Communication Needs Assessment

Please indicate whether the needs listed are:

M = Mandatory
D = Desirable
F = Mandatory in the future (if the PALS [person with ALS]
     deteriorates)
U = Unimportant

Communication Partners	**M**	**D**	**F**	**U**
Does the patient with ALS/MND need to communicate with:				
someone who cannot read (child or nonreader)	☐	☐	☐	☐
someone with no familiarity with the system	☐	☐	☐	☐
someone who has poor vision				
someone who has limited time or patience	☐	☐	☐	☐
someone who does not speak the same language as the patient	☐	☐	☐	☐
someone who is across the room, in another room, or unable to look at a communication board or screen	☐	☐	☐	☐
someone who is not independently mobile	☐	☐	☐	☐
several people at a time (in groups)	☐	☐	☐	☐
someone who is hearing impaired	☐	☐	☐	☐
someone over the phone	☐	☐	☐	☐

Note. Adapted from *Communication Augmentation: A Casebook of Clinical Management* (pp. 209–211), by D. R. Beukelman, K. M. Yorkston, and P. A. Dowden, 1985. San Diego: College-Hill Press. Copyright 1985 by Pro-Ed. Adapted with permission.

Are there any other needs related to
communication partners?

Positioning

	M	D	F	U
Does the patient with ALS/MND need to communicate:				
while walking (carrying a communication system)	☐	☐	☐	☐
with arm slings	☐	☐	☐	☐
upright in bed	☐	☐	☐	☐
on the side in bed	☐	☐	☐	☐
lying flat in bed	☐	☐	☐	☐
in a manually controlled (push) wheelchair	☐	☐	☐	☐
in an electric wheelchair	☐	☐	☐	☐
in an armchair	☐	☐	☐	☐
sitting at a desk	☐	☐	☐	☐

Other Equipment

	M	D	F	U
Does the patient with ALS/MND need to communicate:				
with any type of respiratory equipment	☐	☐	☐	☐

Are there any other needs related to
positioning?

Locations

	M	D	F	U
Does the patient with ALS/MND need to communicate from:				
a single room	☐	☐	☐	☐
multiple rooms within the same building	☐	☐	☐	☐

	M	**D**	**F**	**U**
in dimly lit rooms (i.e., restaurants)	☐	☐	☐	☐
in bright rooms	☐	☐	☐	☐
in noisy rooms	☐	☐	☐	☐
outdoors	☐	☐	☐	☐
while traveling in a car, van, etc.	☐	☐	☐	☐
while moving from place to place within a building	☐	☐	☐	☐
at a desk or computer terminal	☐	☐	☐	☐
in more than two locations in a day	☐	☐	☐	☐

Are there other needs related to locations?

Message Needs	**M**	**D**	**F**	**U**

Does the patient with ALS/MND need to:

	M	**D**	**F**	**U**
call attention	☐	☐	☐	☐
signal emergencies	☐	☐	☐	☐
answer yes/no questions	☐	☐	☐	☐
provide unique information	☐	☐	☐	☐
make requests	☐	☐	☐	☐
carry on a conversation	☐	☐	☐	☐
express emotion	☐	☐	☐	☐
give opinions	☐	☐	☐	☐
convey basic medical needs	☐	☐	☐	☐
greet people	☐	☐	☐	☐
prepare messages in advance	☐	☐	☐	☐
edit texts	☐	☐	☐	☐
edit texts written by others	☐	☐	☐	☐
make changes in diagrams	☐	☐	☐	☐
compile lists	☐	☐	☐	☐
perform calculations	☐	☐	☐	☐
take notes	☐	☐	☐	☐

Are there other needs related to messages?

	M	**D**	**F**	**U**

Message Transmission

Does the patient with ALS/MND need to:

	M	**D**	**F**	**U**
prepare printed messages	☐	☐	☐	☐
prepare spoken messages	☐	☐	☐	☐
talk on the phone	☐	☐	☐	☐
communicate through other equipment (i.e., fax)	☐	☐	☐	☐
communicate privately with some partners	☐	☐	☐	☐
communicate by intercom	☐	☐	☐	☐
communicate via formal letters or reports	☐	☐	☐	☐
communicate on pre-prepared forms	☐	☐	☐	☐
switch from one method of communicating to another during a single communication exchange	☐	☐	☐	☐
communicate in several ways at one time (e.g., taking notes while on the phone)	☐	☐	☐	☐

Are there other needs related to methods of communication?

APPENDIX B

Professional Organizations

ALS Association National Office
21021 Ventura Boulevard, Suite 321, Woodland Hills, CA 91364
Telephone: (818) 340-7500   Fax: (818) 340-2060

National association dedicated to providing information about ALS/MND and research for a cure.

AOTA (American Occupational Therapy Association)
1383 Piccard Drive, P. O. Box 1725, Rockville, MD 20849-1725
Telephone: (301) 729-2682   Fax: (301) 652-7711

National association of occupational therapists, providing information regarding occupational therapists and rehabilitation of patients who are unable to perform activities of daily living.

APA (American Psychological Association)
750 First Street NE, Washington, DC 20002-4242
Telephone: (202) 336-5500

Professional organization for psychologists reflecting ethical and clinical guidelines for researchers and practitioners.

APTA (American Physical Therapy Association)
1111 North Fairfax Street, Alexandria, VA 22314
Telephone: (800) 999-2782; (703) 684-APTA(2782)
Fax: (703) 684-7343

Association providing information to patients with mobility problems and the professionals who treat them (physical therapists & physical therapy assistants).

ASHA (American Speech-Language-Hearing Association)
10801 Rockville Pike, Rockville, MD 20852
Telephone: (301) 897-5700   Fax: (301) 571-0457

National association providing information regarding communication, hearing, and swallowing disorders and the professionals (including speech-language pathologists and audiologists) who diagnose and treat these impairments.

CAMA (Communication Aide Manufacturers Association)
P. O. Box 1039, Evanston, IL 60204-1039
Telephone: (800) 441-2262   Fax: (847) 869-5689

Association representing 18 manufacturers who provide augmentative communication products to nonspeaking patients.

ISAAC (International Society for Augmentative/ Alternative Communication)
P.O. Box 1762 Station R, Toronto, Ontario M4G 4A3, Canada
Telephone: (905) 737-9308   Fax: (905) 737-0624

International association of augmentative communication specialists around the world.

MDA (Muscular Dystrophy Association) National Headquarters
3300 East Sunrise Drive, Tucson, AZ 85718
Telephone: (520) 529-2000   Fax: (520) 529-5454

Association representing the 40 diseases that fall under the category of neuromuscular diseases.

RESNA (Rehabilitation Engineers Society of North America)
1700 N. Moore Street, Suite 1540, Arlington, VA 22209
Telephone: (703) 524-6686   Fax: (703) 524-6630
TTY: (703) 524-6639

National association of rehabilitation engineers.

The Trace Research and Development Center
1500 Highland Avenue, Room S151 Waisman Center,
Madison, WI 53705
Telephone: (608) 262-6966   Fax: (608) 262-8848

Center dedicated to providing comprehensive information on augmentative communication equipment, including software, switches, and so on.

USSAAC (United States Society for Augmentative/ Alternative Communication)
P. O. Box 5271, Evanston, IL 60204-5271
Telephone: (847) 869-2122   Fax: (847) 869-2161

Association representing augmentative communication specialists in the U.S.A.

ON-LINE INTEREST GROUPS AND BULLETIN BOARDS

ALS Interest Group on the Internet
Bob Broedel is the leader of this interest group.
Address: bro@huey.met.fsu.edu

ALS Prodigy Bulletin Board
To access: Hit: "jump"
              Type: medical support
              Type: neurological
              Choose: ALS

APPENDIX C

Funding Resources

The following publications can be obtained by writing or calling CINI directly:

Assistive Technology Funding by Private Health Care Reimbursement Sources, November, 1995.

You've Got To Be Kidding: We Are Not Going To Fund That. (Common Funding "Excuses" Given in Response to Requests for Funding of Computers & Environmental Control Devices), September, 1991.

Common Medicaid Funding "Excuses" for Augmentative and/or Alternative Communication Devices & Services, January, 1995.

You Want Us To Fund That? (Common Funding "Excuses" Given in Response to Requests for Funding of Augmentative Communication Devices & Services), May, 1991.

How to Prepare a Complete Justification for Medicaid Funding of Augmentative Communication Devices & Services, December, 1993.

Survey

In an effort to better meet the needs of the ALS/MND Community, we would like to hear from you. What do you need from a communication resource manual? How would you like the information arranged? Please take a moment to complete the following survey. Once you have had a chance to use the manual, let us know what your needs are.

Name: _____

Address: _____

Telephone Number: _____

Fax: _____

E-mail: _____

Patient:_____   Caregiver:_____   Professional:_____

How often do you expect to refer to this manual? _____

_____

How can this manual better meet your needs? _____

_____

Have you worked with a speech-language pathologist? __

_____

What kind of communication system do you have?_____

_____

What software do you use? _____

_____

How do you access your communication system? _____

_____

Do you use a voice synthesizer? If yes, which one?_____

_____

Do you use an environmental control unit? _____

_____

Where did you hear about CINI or how did you obtain this

resource manual?_____

_____

Additional comments welcomed.
Please write them on the back of this survey.

Please complete and send this survey to:
Communication Independence for the Neurologically Impaired,
   Inc. (CINI)
250 Mercer Street, Suite B1608
New York, NY 10012
Telephone: (516) 874-8354 • Fax: (516) 878-8412

Index

DISCARD